го

MENOPAUSE

BY SALLY FRANZ
ILLUSTRATED BY STEVE MOLLOY

Nightingale Press

an imprint of Wimbledon Publishing Company Ltd.
L O N D O N

First published in Great Britain
by Wimbledon Publishing Co. Ltd
London P.O. Box 9779 SW19 7ZG

ISBN: 1 903222 38 9

Produced in Great Britain
Printed and bound in Hungary

BABY BOOMERS

Baby Boomers are everywhere. In the beginning they filled some seventy million baby strollers, then millions of dance halls doing the Lindy Hop and the Twist. At college they filled millions of administration buildings, usually in protest about how hard their life had been this far. Let's face it, they're probably the biggest group of babies the world has ever known. I should know, I'm one of them!

...And whingers. We have taken complaining to a new level. My parents were middle class, so, of course, I had to denounce them as capitalist pigs (right after they paid for my clothes, car and tuition).

I grew up under a government which guaranteed

civil liberties and freedom of speech, so I used my freedom to drop out and criticize.

Inevitably, the fire of youth gradually burned out and, somewhere along the way, my life of dissolution turned into management, mortgages and materialism.

But then something even more horrible happened - I turned forty and became part of the *older generation*.

Dealing with the horror of becoming my own parents hasn't been easy. But Baby Boomers are good at re-inventing themselves. In fact, we invented the term 're-inventing yourself'!

Now we are having to admit to ourselves that we might just be able to trust someone over we might just be able to trust someone over thirty, or forty or fifty or, God help us, sixty! And as these rules change we find that life goes on. Though not without a few more obstacles to overcome…

So with all the enthusiasm of hurling oneself in protest over a police barrier, we strike out to the new frontiers of life as mature (or at least wrinkled) Baby Boomers.

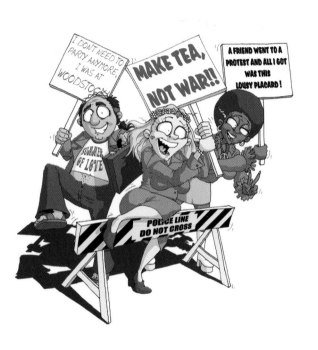

INTRODUCTION TO THE MENOPAUSE

There are at least fifty million female Baby Boomers wandering around the free world - every one of them just a few grams short of oestrogen. They have just figured out they've had 30% less salary than their male counterparts for the last thirty years, not to mention never having received a penny for decades of housework. Now somebody *is* going to pay!

The menopause is when your 'friend' stops visiting. You know, that punctual little fellow who never failed to bring a basket of goodies for you each month - headaches, cramps, nausea, fainting, tears, mood swings. It's like Christmas with your mother-in-law ... every twenty eight days!

Now all that is about to change. That 'friend' is about to get cut off. And, instead of being knocked down every month with a case of the female flu, these women are going to get stronger and stronger. They are going to ROAR. They are going to take control of their lives and have the things they deserve ... after they've crossed just one last little bridge - the *menopause*.

The problem with the menopause is that your 'friend' doesn't just stop calling one day and that's that. No, *this* friend is like an ex-boyfriend that won't take a hint. This friend stops by, disappears, stops by again unannounced and then forgets to call for a month or two. This can go on for - well, you tell me how long it takes to get rid of a bad relationship? We could be talking five years or more.

The menopause has all the symptoms of your 'friend' in a really bad mood: severe cramps, more than one visit a month, acne, irritability, early ageing symptoms, weight fluctuations, forgetfulness and, well, there are quite a few more surprises to tackle before you are in the clear.

The good news is you are not alone and you are not going crazy. Okay, you *might* be going crazy, but you are definitely not alone!

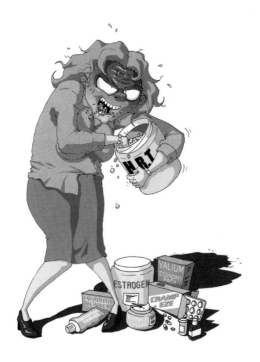

IDENTIFYING
THE MENOPAUSAL
BABY BOOMER

THE MAN-EATER

She has an insatiable appetite for younger men:
the paper boy, the lawn boy, the altar boy.
She orders pizza three times a day just
to leer at the delivery boy.

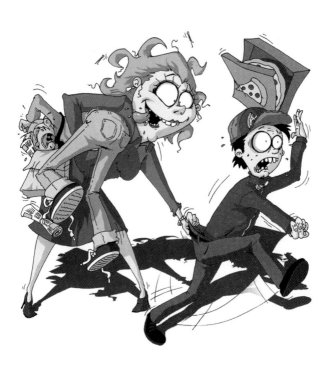

THE BINGER

This menopausal women will eat anything in sight.
She would sell her first born for a cheesecake
and her beloved poodle for a family box of
chocolates. She's already pawned her communion
cross for a tin of butter cookies and traded in
her husband for a side-by-side refrigerator.

THE MAN-HATER

Ever since her husband ran off with his young secretary, she's had it in for men. The man-hater will punish you for the sins of her husband, her father and her boss. A date with her is like taking a wrong turn into a bad neighbourhood and finding it's a deadend. Or like kissing the White Witch of Narnia square on the lips.

THE NEUROTIC

No incident is too small for her to have a breakdown in public. She cries when she misses a parking spot, sees a puppy in distress, or gets caught with eleven items in the ten item row. She keeps a box of Kleenex by the TV to dry her eyes during all those old films. Funny though, *Conan the Barbarian* never used to set her off like this.

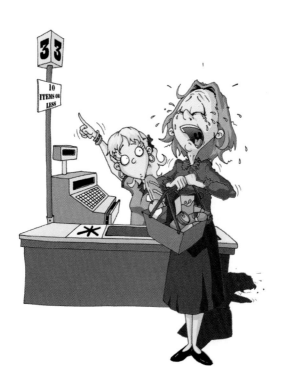

THE NARCISSIST

She's had it nipped, tucked and sand-blasted.
Every inch of her is tighter than clingfilm on a
pork chop. Her teeth are capped, her hair is
tinted. She doesn't look old, she doesn't look
young … she looks like worn sheets that have
been starched, ironed and stretched on an over-
sized mattress. One wrong move and the whole
enchilada will tear from stem to stern.

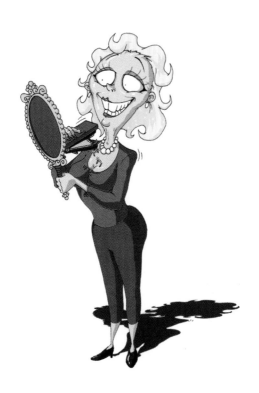

THE SPEED QUEEN

If you're quick, you'll catch a glance of this creature careering down the street: mobile phone in one hand, lipstick in the other, brain on hold. She weaves through police barriers like an Olympic slalom skier. She thinks an empty pavement is an overtaking lane. She believes the amber light means 'go like a bat out of hell'. She only brakes for small animals and shoe sales.

THE FEMINIST

She insists on opening her own doors, thank you very much. She'll pick up the bill. She'll unblock the sink. She'll manage the children. She'll plan and pay for the trips. But don't even think about lending a hand. Complaining she has to do all the work is what makes it all worthwhile.

THE OVER-HEATER

It's not the fountain of youth soaking those bed sheets! If you want to know if she is having hot flushes, just check the thermostat: the heat will be turned off in January, yet the room will be like a jungle. She can generate enough heat to barbecue a steak over her chest.

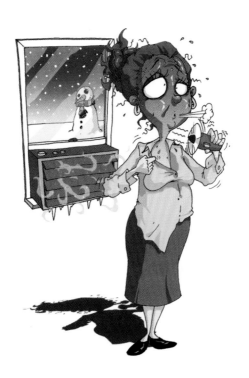

THE PARANOIAC

She suspects everybody of being after her.
The gasman is changing the meter to charge her
more. The butcher has loaded scales to cheat her.
Do not let her near wicker chairs in pantyhose -
snagged stockings are a part of her conspiracy
theory against women. She is convinced her cat
likes the neighbour best. Maybe the cat has a point.

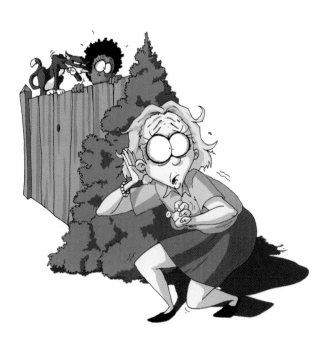

THE SCATTER-BRAIN

She has lost her car keys, hair brush and glasses six times this week and it's only Tuesday. She made the check-out girl at the local store call the police because her wallet was stolen, only to find it on the coffee table at home. The doctor gave her a jar of *gingko biloba* to improve her memory, but she can't remember where she put it.

THE FLAKER

She has skin so dry that she looks like a souvenir plastic snow globe whenever she moves. She is peeling like paint off an old house. The good news? She figures at this rate she'll lose ten pounds a year through shedding alone.

THE SNAPPER

She wasn't much fun when she was young, but an absence of oestrogen has taken her to new levels of irritation. Now she's MEAN. She yells at children, kicks kittens and parks in handicapped parking spots. Somebody ought to stop her! Somebody wearing a steel box and a hockey mask.

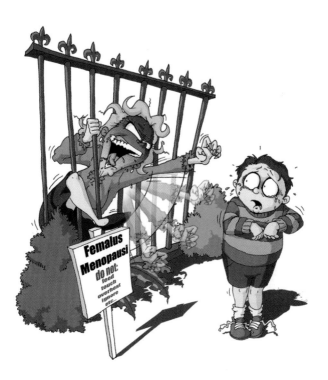

THE DEPRESSIVE

You come home to find the water has been running in the sink since breakfast. She's sitting in a chair looking out into space. She is in her well, with nothing worth wishing for, right at the bottom. She's convinced this is the last day of her life. You must pry open her mouth and insert vast quantities of chocolate.

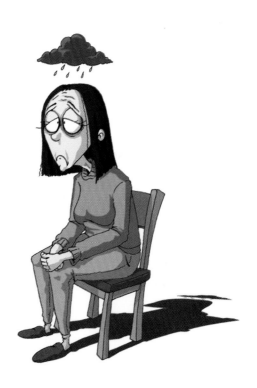

THE BLOATER

What's round and soft and sensitive to the touch?
What *isn't*? Ankles, arms, face, feet, fingers ... and
don't even think about touching her breasts,
they're off-limits until further notice. On the bright
side, living with water retention has an element of
mystery - you never know if you're going to wake
up looking like Twiggy or Miss Piggy.

THE MOOD SWINGER

Up, down, back and forth - this gal puts the 'fun' in dysfunctional. One day she thinks you're clever, the next you're disgusting. One day you're witty the next you're insipid. You never know where you stand with her, so you'd better stand at a distance.

THE SELF-RIGHTEOUS

Hell hath no fury like a woman saved. Her sins have been forgiven and forgotten, forever. Yours, on the other hand, are grist for the judgment mill. She is suddenly against sex, alcohol, cigarettes, bad language and loud music. Now if she could just scrub her name and number off the back wall at Murphy's pub from last month...

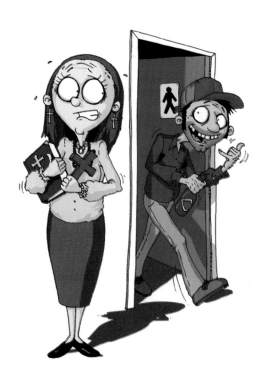

THE SHOP-A-HOLIC

Down goes the oestrogen level, up goes the
credit card debt. So many sales, such little time.
She has seven novelty tin openers, three rolling
pins, four blenders, five egg racks. After all, you
never know when you might need a spare. She
buys clothes in sizes too small - just in case she
gets a tape worm and ends up a size six!

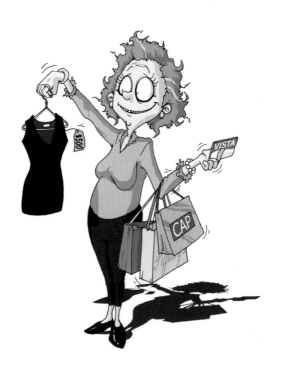

THE HERBALIST

She has a homemade recipe for everything.
Depressed? St. John's Wort. Bloated? Sassafras tea.
Short on oestrogen? Yam cream. Moody?
Lemongrass pie. In fact, if you just graze alongside
her cow you should be fine (you do have four
stomachs don't you?)

THE CASH MACHINE

She likes to throw money at problems. That
usually makes them go away. It worked with the
last three husbands, her failing business and her
annoying relatives. Now she is shopping for
someone to ease her menopausal strife. The
Valentine's day Porsche she bought her plastic
surgeon should do the trick.

THE RE-ARRANGER

You come home at night to find your furniture is completely changed around. And she lives next door. If she gets upstairs she'll feng shui your underwear drawer. If you are what you eat, you're a bean curd … she's replaced all your animal products with tofu substitute. She's obsessed with helping you - and she *will* help you … right into the arms of your therapist.

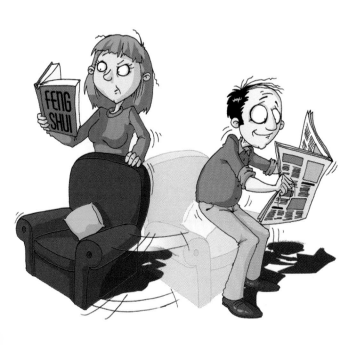

IDENTIFYING
THE CALL OF THE
MENOPAUSE

'Is it hot in here,
or is it just me?'

(Overheard in a sauna at the gym.)

'I am sick and tired
of serving other people. Get
your own damn meal!'

(Most often uttered by Baby Boomer
air-stewardesses at 30,000 feet.)

'Why am I halfway down
the stairs? Oh well, I'm
almost to the kitchen. I'll
snack until I remember.'

(2 am.)

'I'm not crying because
I'm sad, I'm crying because
I'm happy.'

(Then two seconds later: 'I'm not laughing
because I'm happy, I'm laughing because
the pain is too great to cry'.)

'Dye it, streak it, perm it,
fluff it - you know make it
look natural.'

(To her hairdresser.)

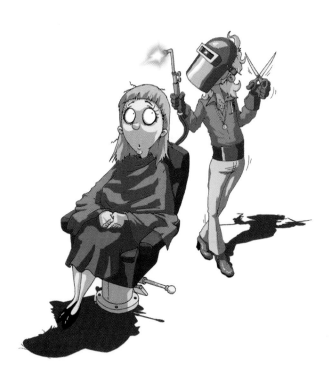

'Upset? No! Why
do you ask?'

(Release her grip from your throat
before attempting a response.)

'I am mad as hell and
I am not going to take it
any more.'

(Usually spoken to the cash machine
as it refuses to hand out cash!)

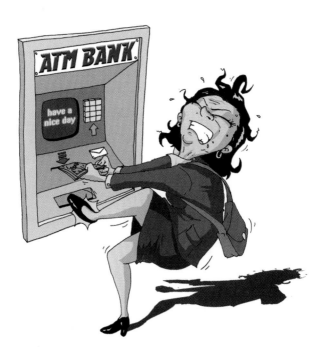

'No, I don't want you to understand. All I want is for you to get the flu, jungle virus, migraine headaches, and arthritis all at once and then I'll ask YOU what's for dinner.'

(Every night at home.)

'I am not hormonal, you are being unreasonable!'

(Spoken to her computer.)

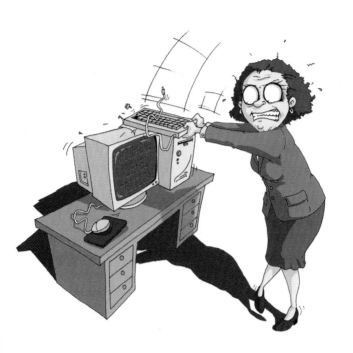

'Honestly,
I never saw it.'

(Said of any obstacle that meets with her car's back
bumper in the shopping centre car park.)

'I feel like a teenager again:
acne, low self-esteem, no
plans for the future,
slumped shoulders, awkward
around the opposite sex,
craving snack food and
wanting someone to blame.'

(Said to a complete stranger in an elevator.)

'You're awfully cute,
want to come up and
see my etchings?'

(Said to the boy scout who just
helped her across the street.)

'Pump it up! Pump it!
Pump up the volume!'

(Said to the plastic surgeon as he
injects the collagen.)

'I don't care what it costs,
just get rid of these wrinkles!'

(Overheard at the dry cleaners and
the cosmetics counter.)

'These are perfect;
I'll take them!'

(Spoken as she purchases a pair of shoes
she knows she will never wear again.)

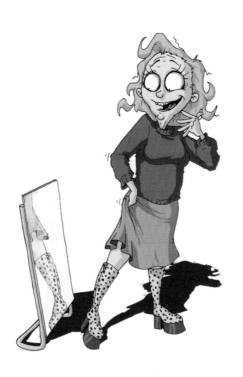

'I can't wear these tights they're ruined! Just look at these ladders and snags!'

(Spoken looking at her bare legs without her glasses on.)

'Someone has stolen my car. Help! Police! Oh never mind, there it is.'

(Spoken while standing in her own driveway.)

'Half-duck and half-beaver? I can beat that: crow's feet, turkey wattle, pigeon toes, rhino haunches and alligator skin.'

(Spoken to the duck-billed platypus at the zoo.)

'I'm going for a walk
to calm down.'

(Last seen a week ago on the A1,
heading north.)

'You never listen to me!'

(Shouted at her therapist.)

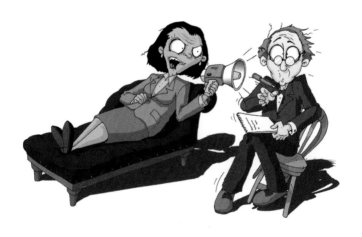

AUNT SASSY'S ADVICE PAGES

Aunt Sassy does not suffer fools gladly. Her advice pages are filled with vitriol and venom. What else would you expect from a menopausal sage? She knows all about hormones, mood swings and hot flushes. And what she doesn't know, she makes up.

You got a problem with that?

I didn't think so.

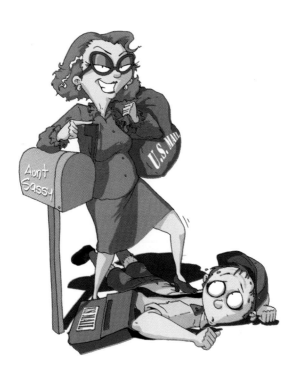

Dear Aunt Sassy,

I think my very own mother is becoming menopausal. She yells about the mess all the time, especially when she comes home from work, and when she's not yelling, she's crying. What do you think?

Confused in Colchester

Dear Confused,

Let's review the situation. Every day your mother works eight hours at the office and eight hours at home. You and your friends keep her up the rest of the time, so she's clearly exhausted and deprived of sleep. Let's try a little experiment: why not get a haircut, wear proper clothes and find a well-paid job, offer to pay for and cook dinner, clean-up after yourself and mop the kitchen floor once in a while, if only because your friends seem to get stuck to it right in front of the fridge. If Mum is still angry after all that, well then, she *may* be menopausal.

Your ever-doting,

AUNT SASSY

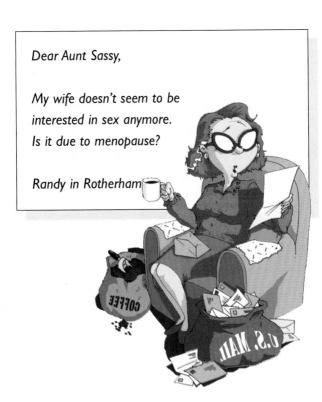

Dear Randy,

Often a fluctuation in hormones *does* impact
the level of desire a woman experiences.
Far greater than the hormones, though, is the 'over-
hang factor'. As in 'just how far does your gut hang
over your jeans'?

For too long bad sex has been blamed on menopausal
women. Lack of performance in men is rarely due to
a lack of proper enticement from women. *You* must
entice as well. It's hard to get geared up for Don Juan
when all that shows up is the Taco Bell Chihuahua.

Remember: after-shave and deodorant after a bath,
not instead of. And also, if your foreplay can be timed
with an egg timer you're not doing it correctly.

Passionately yours,

AUNT SASSY

Dear Aunt Sassy,

Help! I am four different sizes in one day, due to water-retention. I go from thin to fat in ten seconds. What can I do?

Fluctuating in Farnham

Dear Fluctuating,

Many menopausal women change sizes faster than they change their minds. The key is to wear clothes that expand like an accordion and can snap back like a soldier to attention. Here's a quick list of outfits that expand as you do: kilts with lots of folds and pleats; double-breasted jackets that can become single-breasted; any dress with a large scarf (to hide a zipper that has had to be undone); ponchos in interesting fabrics (steer clear of horizontal stripes, large checks and anything that looks like sofa material or the back-seat of a 1950s sedan); cardigan sweaters to tie around your waist (and hide unbuttoned waist bands.)

Alternatively, you could just cover everything up with fifty four inch jeans and a knee-length T-shirt. Better to be 'phat' than fat anyday!

Fashionably yours,

AUNT SASSY

Dear Aunt Sassy,

I keep losing my keys and glasses. If I lose my glasses first I can't see to find my keys. If I lose my keys first I can't get in the house where my second pair of glasses are.

Lost in Luton

Dear Lost,

Memory loss is one of the first signs of menopause. We just have to do our best until the oestrogen pills kick in - after all, ladies of culture and status know that composure is paramount.

We don't want to be caught loitering shiftily in our own front gardens waiting for someone to come back and let us in, do we? Of course not, so why not attach your frames to one of those lovely chain necklaces sold at fine petrol stations everywhere? The nine carat gold will bring out the green in your dimming eyes.

For the keys, well, middle-aged folks often hide a spare set in places they know no-one will look: under the doormat, for instance, or beneath the loose stone on the pathway. Failing that, try the 'brick through the window' routine and blame it on 'menopausal tension'. You think anyone's going to argue with you in this mood?

Insightfully yours,

AUNT SASSY

GUIDELINES
FOR HANDLING
THE MENOPAUSAL
WOMAN

■   *Don't bring home leftovers and expect to see them again, they are considered public domain to be taxed at will.*

■ *Don't defend yourself, especially when you are right - just say, "I'm so sorry!" (Also, "you're right, I see your side of it, I was wrong.") In fact, just start with those phrases when you get up in the morning as a pre-emptive strike.*

■ *Don't bring home copies of Smash Hits, or those Calvin Klein ads. She is only human. (Definitely no posters of Ronan Keating.)*

■ *Don't ever tell her she has too many shoes (Or clothes, candles, cushions on the bed etc.)*

■ *Never ever answer the question: do I look fat to you? (Especially if she is cooking with hot oil and sharp knives.)*

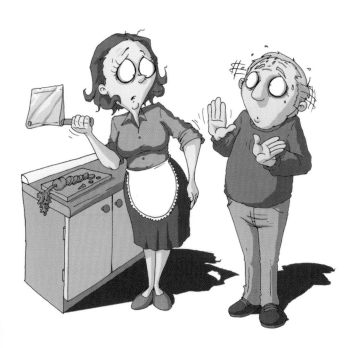

■   When the car comes home dented assume it was a 'hit and run' and happened in the car park. (Look, you're lucky she even remembered where the car was parked!)

■   Put a limit on all credit cards when she is particularly hormonal.

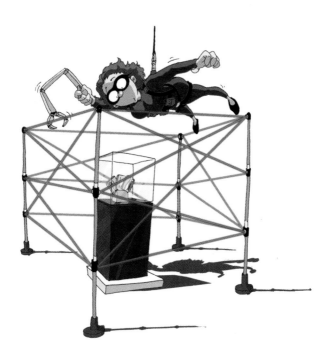

■ *If her self-esteem is wavering and she asks, "Do you still love me?" the answer is YES. (I don't care if she looks like the Michelin tyre guy in drag, has more chest hair than Tarzan and more mood swings than the Flying Wallendas at a three ring circus ... the answer is YES!)*

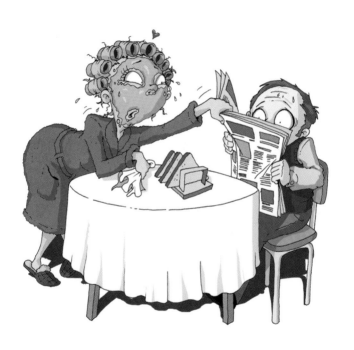

■ *If she asks "Is it hot in here?" The answer is YES. (I don't care if you're feeding ice cream to eskimos - the answer is YES!)*

■ *If her skin is flakey and she asks, "Is it dry in here?" The answer is YES. (I don't care if it has rained for forty days and nights and the animals are lining up two-by-two in your backyard - the answer is YES!)*

■ *WHY? Because it is a simple fact that women who are low on oestrogen are also high on adrenaline. And that means she can hurt you!*

CONCLUSION

Are you moody and irritable? Is your body expanding faster than a hot air balloon under a burner? Have you lost a set of car keys each week for the past six months? YES! After thirty years of surviving cyclic biological problems you've discovered it was all just preparation for the Armageddon of hormone battles.

The menopause is a test. It is one of life's most gruelling training courses and it comes at the end of life, not at twenty, when you might have had the energy for it.

Why were we not warned about this? Was I the only one who envisioned my waning years to be one long Edith Wharton Victorian garden party? You know, lovely clean grandchildren dressed in white sailor suits pushing toy boats across the pond; ever-blooming weed-free gardens spilling over onto Thomas Kincade paintings of thatched roof cottages; and rolling white clouds. Wasn't I supposed to get a rest from all this hormone nonsense and become a handsome, good-tempered matron? I *can* look pretty good if I get some rest once in a while.

But alas, it is not to be. My once-smooth skin looks like folds of organza on a debutante's skirt. I'm drying up and overheating. The garden of my autumn years looks more like the Sahara. And my grandchildren look like hookers and bikers. My reward for surviving thirty years of monthly hardship is that my hormones have become the focus of my life.

The menopause is like completing a five day dance marathon, only to find out that the first prize is a lifetime certificate for more dance lessons.

So what about the men? What are they to do as the women in their lives go through this horror? They cannot pretend to understand what is happening. They have never cramped, fainted, bled and still got to work on time. They have never carried and delivered a baby while trying to keep an entire family up-and-running. And they have certainly never had to sit under a hot hair dryer for three hours for the perm to 'take' because hormones have left their hair too limp to be seen in public.

One brave and honest man once said, "There is one thing you have to know about the battle of the sexes: men do not win the battle, they are permitted to live".

So, here's my advice: women, remember that you are strong. You *will* pull through because the human race is counting on you to get back on your feet and set an example. Men, be willing to go through menopause *with* your woman, not against her. Be there for her when she needs you. Rub her feet or her back, *don't* rub her the wrong way. Remember, if you're kind, generous and forgiving she will reward you one day by being kind to you in your old age. If not, you may not make it to old age!